USMLE STEP 2 CK & 3: CARDIOLOGY

The Titanium Series

BY FAIZ ANAND, MD

Table of Contents

Table of Contents

CARDIOLOGY
The Titanium Series

INTRODUCTION

How do I navigate the cardiology portion of the USMLE exams?

- Cardiology is one of the most important sections of the exam. As a rule, exam questions are prioritized in a manner that appropriately represents diagnosis found in the real world [e.g. MI (myocardial infarction), angina, CHF (congestive heart failure), DM (diabetes mellitus), HTN (hypertension), asthma, COPD (chronic obstructive pulmonary disease) and pneumonia are high-yield topics]

- The cardiology section should be reviewed more times than any other section. Know it by heart and understand the key steps in therapeutic management. Also, repeat the commercially available question banks until you perform well above the average score. Unfortunately, question banks do not translate to actual scores in the exam, but failing to complete the questions may translate into suboptimal performance on the exam. Thus, it is in your best interest to be on equal footing with other students. Finish the banks, twice – Do not simply go through the motions when you attempt to answer the questions for the second time (chances are you've probably memorized it). Instead, try to work your way through the logic that let you arrive at the answer to begin with. Read all the commentary including the explanations for all the incorrect choices. The explanations for the wrong choices contain 'factoids' that provide the foundation for future questions. Try to get into the head of the exam content creator(s). Why are certain lab values introduced in the vignette? Do they serve as distractors or relevant pieces of information? Of course, it goes without saying that you should not delve into any question (during your preparation or the actual exam day) beyond a reasonable amount of time. This is not a philosophy exam. *The Titanium Series: Cardiology* is designed to allow students to reach their peak performance on the exam. It is written for both novice and advanced test takers alike. It is not meant to be a comprehensive review on the subject, but aims to provide the necessary tools to "own" the cardiology section of the exam.

Chapter 1: Conceptualizing Shock

It's been an annual tradition for the exam content creators to reintroduce a table describing the parameters for the different types of shock. You might see one of these questions testing your understanding of shock. Perhaps, even two (if you are lucky). These questions may appear intimidating at first but are fairly easy to answer if you've memorized a table or if you have a basic understanding of the relationship governing Resistance and C.O (cardiac output).

What is shock?

In order to understand shock, you have to be able to visualize the process. No need for complex diagrams. At the most basic level, a flow diagram for shock can be summarized by the following equation:

Shock -> Hypoxia

Shock is a pathological medical condition that is the direct result of hypoxia. As a clinician, you are attempting to relieve the hypoxia (before it progresses to irreversible cellular or tissue damage). Lets take a look at an expanded flow diagram:

Shock -> [blood perfusion error] -> Hypoxia

Blood perfusion is responsible for delivering oxygen to the body's cells and tissues.

Signs and Symptoms

- Confusion or altered mental status (not enough blood flow/oxygen to brain)
- Tachycardia (reflexive in nature – the body is attempting to compensate or correct for the acute changes)
- Excessive sweating (reflexive or compensatory in nature)
- Decreased urine output (the body is attempting to compensate by conserving volume)
- Elevated BUN and Creatinine [(BUN and Creatinine tend to have a directly proportional relationship but there are cases of isolated increases in BUN or Creatinine – regardless, these values suggest a problem at the systemic level, notably, the kidneys) (in healthy humans, the kidneys receive a whopping 25% of C.O)]
- Low BP (reduced oxygen delivery to tissues, in particular, hypovolemic shock)
- Diminished pulse (more or less universal amongst the types of shocks, namely, anaphylactic, distributive, endocrine, hemorrhagic, hypovolemic, neurogenic, obstructive, septic, traumatic etc.)

An important parameter that we look at in shock is Pulmonary Capillary Wedge Pressure or PCWP*. It can be elevated or suppressed in shock. It could also be normal. As far as the exam is concerned, the clinicians aim to maintain a PCWP of 12-14 via fluid therapy. Fluid therapy is the primary step in the management of shock.

*Equivalent abbreviations include PCWP=PWP=PAWP=PVWP=PAOP

Fluid therapy can be augmented by administration of packed red blood cells (PRBCs) as necessitated by the situation at hand. If the bleeding does not subside, administer PRBCs. If the laboratory values

6

indicate anemia, administer PRBCs. Further management includes the administration of vasopressors, generally in a stepwise manner.

Now, back to the question that I've mentioned earlier. In order to answer the question, we need to be mindful of the arrows. It is a game of arrows. There are 3 metrics [(PCWP, C.O and Systemic Vascular Resistance (SVR)]. For the sake of simplicity, I will refer to PCWP as "P" for pressure and SVR as "R" for resistance). C.O is inversely proportional to "R" (when the CO goes downhill, the "R" goes uphill and vice versa). Likewise, the C.O is also inversely proportional to "P" (when the CO goes uphill, the "P" goes downhill and vice versa, except for hypovolemia—There is simply not enough volume to account for "P").

Anaphylactic Shock vs. Septic Shock

The parameters are exactly the same (in some cases, a septic shock patient may yield a normal "P") but the management is different. You begin treating the patient by employing general guidelines for managing shock. The next step would require that you tailor the treatment to take into consideration the Anaphylaxis (a combo of epinephrine and steroid) state and the Septic (give antibiotic as sepsis is often the direct result of a bacterial infection) shock state.

In both cases, the C.O ↑ and the "R" ↓
In both cases, the heart is pumping overtime to fight the ongoing sepsis or anaphylaxis.

Cardiogenic Shock vs. Tamponade Shock

In terms of pathophysiology, these are different entities that require tailored treatments following the general guidelines for managing shock.

Both types of shock profiles employ the same metrics, namely:

P ↑ C.O↓ R ↑

However, the mainstay of pericardial tamponade therapy involves administration of the oxygen (to address the hypoxia and shortness of breath), monitoring and pericardiocentesis (definitive therapy).

Alternatively, a thoracotomy can be performed, but it is invasive and not the best answer choice.

Likewise, the mainstay of cardiogenic shock involves administration of oxygen. You are still responsible for initiating fluid and vasopressor therapy as it is essential for the management of alleviating any shock state. A cardiogenic shock is a pump failure. It is not surprising that the C.O is abysmally low, as the heart's pumping mechanism has been jeopardized.

The inotropic and vasopressor agents are used in the hopes of augmenting the heart's natural capacity to pump blood. However, this is often not sufficient and an intra-aortic balloon pump or similar devices are installed to facilitate the reduction of workload for the heart. Ultimately, the patient may need to undergo aortic valve replacement or even a cardiac transplantation.

Hypovolemic Shock

How do you correct hypovolemic shock? The same way you address shock, in general. Therapy for hypovolemic shock does not need to be tailored.

P ↓ C.O↓ R ↑

All of the arrows point down, except "R" –if the vascular resistance was down as well, then the patient would be dead. C.O is low because there is really not that much volume to distribute.

Patients with massive pulmonary embolism will exhibit diminished C.O coupled with a rise in vascular resistance. However, the "P" will be normal, as far as the exam is concerned. It involves a different pathophysiological mechanism altogether; the patient will require thrombolysis (as well as the default shock protocol). If the patient is a poor candidate for therapy by means of thrombolysis, arrange for surgical removal of the embolus.

Chapter 2: Heart Murmurs

I would advise memorizing the list of heart murmurs (attributes, quality, location etc.) and the techniques that amplify or diminish the murmurs (e.g. handgrip/valsalva/standing/squatting/inspiration/exhalation). This is one of the sections of the exam that can be memorized directly or understood intuitively (or both). It is best to learn them closer to the exam date as they tend to leverage the test takers short-term memory. A number of perennial exam favorites include, HOCM, MVP (mid-systolic click) PDA (e.g. continuous machine-like murmur) and ASD (wide-fixed split).

Do not confuse a "pericardial rub" with "pericardial knocking". It is a relatively common mistake. Pericardial rub are audible heart sounds that are characteristic of pericarditis, a condition in which there is an inflamed (but, not fibrotic) pericardium. Pericardial knock are audible heart sounds that are characteristic of constrictive pericarditis, a condition in which there is an inflamed **and** fibrotic pericardium (will be visible on CXR). The etiologies and therapeutic management of these conditions are distinct. Non-complicated cases of pericarditis can be managed by ASA or NSAIDS. Pericarditis is readily identified on EKG because of its characteristic (diffuse) ST segment elevation +/- PR segment depression.

Constrictive pericarditis is a more severe condition with increased mortality. The therapeutic intervention of choice is pericardial stripping. Patients with long-standing constrictive pericarditis may demonstrate low voltage QRS on the EKG. Any restrictive (i.e.

constricting) condition (infiltrating or otherwise) may dampen QRS readings on EKG.

Conditions with low voltage QRS include: Schleroderma (of the heart), Myxodema (infiltrative), Amyloidosis (infiltrative), Hemochromatosis (infiltrative), Sarcoidosis (infiltrative) and Pericardial Effusion (constrictive effect; limits size of pericardial cavity).

A low voltage EKG reading will look something like this:

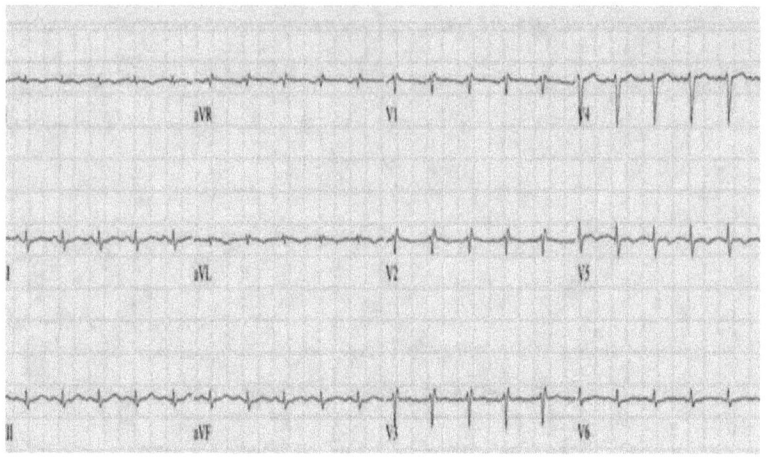

If you have additional time (always a good thing!), learn about the snaps, heaves and lifts as they relate to various heart sounds –they are somewhat lower yield. Constrictive pericarditis is responsible (in a manner similar to tamponade and various pericardial disease entities) for hemodynamic changes. These hemodynamic changes have a tangible effect on blood pressure. The patient may exhibit a paradoxical pulse (*pulsus paradoxus*) while inspiring, leading to a precipitous drop in blood pressure (e.g. 10 mm Hg +).

A paradoxical pulse tends to go hand in hand with a cardiac tamponade as an inbuilt property of the Beck's Triad* or the first component of the triad.

*Beck's Triad
1. Low BP
2. JVP (distended neck veins)
3. Distant (muffled heart sounds).

A paradoxical pulse** can be associated with pulmonary embolism (and/or massive PE), hypovolemic shock as pronounced hemodynamic changes can be found in these conditions. However, *Pulsus paradoxus* isn't a specific trait of any the aforementioned disease entities. It can also be present in the following conditions:

- Sleep apnea
- Asthma
- COPD
- Pericarditis
- Laryngotracheobronchitis

**Pulsus Paradoxus is defined as a drop in systolic blood pressure of >10 mmHg that accompanies inspiration. The word, 'paradoxus' or 'paradoxical' is a bit of a misnomer as it is not inversely proportional to the rise in systolic pressure. Furthermore, the phenomenon occurs independently of heart rate (pulse). For reference, note that baseline conditions involve a drop in systolic pressure of < 10 mm Hg that accompanies inspiration.*

Pulses and Medical Signs

The exam wants you to be familiar with a number of pulse types. In typical fashion, they may opt to describe the pulse rather than using the medical names that you have been ingrained with in your head. That's why it is far better to know that a 'slow riding pulse' is associated with Aortic stenosis rather than the knee-jerk (sorry for the medical pun) recall that 'pulsus tardus' is associated with Aortic stenosis. This logic is fairly consistent across the exam; a number of concepts and terms are briefly described in the vignette as opposed to throwing around buzzwords. The exam tests your understanding of medical knowledge more than your ability to recall or dependence on memory. Likewise, ordinary and suboptimal test takers would readily **associate** 'pulsus alternans' with left ventricular dysfunction. Advanced test takers will **understand** that pulsus alternans indicates a severely compromised ejection fraction (as a function of a dysfunctional left ventricle) and that there are reduced stroke volumes and a poor prognostic outcome. However, don't get carried away and attempt to learn all the physiology. Cardiology is vast. It's about striking the right balance. You only need a few points here and there, enough to understand a concept. And, you need to stay focused. Excessive information can also get in the way and cause you to go astray. Apply efficient test-taking strategies and stay focused (refer to appendix for examples of efficient test-taking strategies).

Watson's water hammer pulse and Corrigan's collapsing pulse are familiar terms from medical school. They are not common medical signs in the real world but have been described in the medical literature due to their *classic* and memorable nature. These are not two separate pulses but merely two names for the same pulse phenomena found in aortic regurgitation (aortic insufficiency) or AR. All this really means is that there is a forceful/ rebounding/widened pulse

14

associated with an elevated stroke volume (emanating from the left ventricle) resulting from the presence of an insufficient aortic valve. Aortic insufficiency (aortic regurgitation) is a leaky aortic valve with a reduction in elastic properties and concomitant dilatation at the level of the aortic root.

Lastly, let's take a look at *pulsus tardus* or the slow-rising pulse (*anacrotic* pulse). It's found in aortic valve stenosis (AS) and is pretty much the opposite of what you find in AR (e.g. Corrigan's pulse). Remember that the Corrigan's pulse is robust and forceful. In contrast, the pulsus tardus is faint and small. Aortic valve stenosis (AS) is generally associated with narrow pulse pressure (as opposed to AR which has widened pulse pressure). It's probably a good idea to apply heuristics* during your exam preparation schedule. It might be a good idea to visualize the AR as having a valve that is "floppy/leaky" (insufficient) and AS having a valve that is "tightened" (stenotic). In that sense it is much more easier to navigate the cardiology section of the exam if we stick to basic valve properties and functionality. In the AR, the pulse is widened because the valve is floppy. In the AS, the pulse is narrowed because the valve is tightened or stenotic. It's not entirely accurate as a clinical concept, but heuristics will allow you to navigate the exam and effectively allows for a "personalized" approach to understanding valve function [e.g. Ejection Fraction (EF), valve area and LV end systolic dimension].

What is a Heuristic?

According to Merriam-Webster online dictionary:

Heuristic: "involving or serving as an aid to learning, discovery, or problem-solving by experimental and especially trial-and-error methods heuristic techniques a heuristic assumption; also: of or relating to exploratory problem-solving techniques that utilize self-educating techniques to improve performance".

Heuristics serve as an invaluable tool for consolidating large volumes of clinical information.

Chapter 3: Valvular Deficits

<u>Mitral Valve Prolapse (MVP)</u>

MVP is a benign condition that may result from myxomatous degeneration* of the valve and is regarded as a precursor for mitral regurgitation (MR). In the exam, you will likely receive a vignette of a woman that is under 35 years of age with a chief complaint of intermittent palpitations and/or non-severe chest pain. In real life, this is debatable, and the Framingham Heart Study did not yield any disparities across male or female subjects. In the past, USMLE exams associated MVP with panic disorder. This is not the case in newer editions of the exam. Having said this, it is possible to find this condition within the context of underlying anxiety. The patient is having anxiety because she is concerned that her symptoms (e.g. palpitations, chest pain, tachycardia) might be serious. They are not. As a clinician, you are required to provide symptomatic treatment. You have to address the chest pain, tachycardia, shortness of breath, anxiety or whatever else issues the patient may present with. A beta-blocker is sufficient therapy for symptom resolution. If the patient presents to the office for a general health assessment and a mid systolic click (or late systolic murmur) is discovered incidentally, provide reassurance and move on.

We do not treat asymptomatic conditions. There are only a handful of asymptomatic conditions (e.g. those that involve worsening prognosis if left untreated) on the exam that need to be addressed promptly. <u>All valvular dysfunctions (as well as ejection fractions) are best visualized by echocardiogram (ultrasound of the heart).</u> For example, an echocardiogram is performed if the clinician suspects a valve rupture (or even, a septum or wall rupture, for that matter); definitive treatment necessitates surgical repair.

Mitral Regurgitation (MR)

Remember, a "regurgitation" or "insufficiency" basically means that the valve is floppy or wider than baseline (as opposed to stenotic conditions such as MS and AS). What could compromise the integrity of the valve? One possibility is an insult to the Chordae Tendineae— these are flexible supporting structures (cords) that direct the opening (and, closing) of the mitral valve. Can you imagine why broken cords would lead to an "insufficient" valve? Bacterial endocarditis or valvular infiltrates of any kind [e.g. Non-bacterial thrombotic endocarditis (marantic/verrucous/Libman-Sacks)] can influence the overall morphology of the valves. Patients present to the ER with shortness of breath (SOB); as a side note to this information, dyspnea can have either a cardiac or pulmonary origin. Chronic MR (or superimposed Pulmonary HTN or asymptomatic MR with low EF) needs to be surgically addressed.

Treatment (definitive): **Mitral Valve Repair or Mitral Valve Replacement**

Mitral Stenosis (MS)

What causes MS? The majority of patients with MS will have a past medical history of a rheumatic fever event. Rheumatic fever occurs 3 weeks (+/- 1 week) after an infection with streptococcal throat infection; symptomatic MS may develop 30-50 years after the infection. Less frequently, MR and AR are associated with a history of rheumatic fever. The key to navigating the MS section is having a sense of imagination. You will need to fully appreciate the

18

relationship between form and function. Morphological changes in anatomy will go hand in hand with the symptoms experienced by the patient. A few paragraphs down the line, I will describe the relevant concepts (e.g. form vs. function) that you will be expected to know for this particular murmur.

MS could also develop in a previously asymptomatic patient during the course of pregnancy (remember, there are morphological changes taking place during pregnancy with increased pressure on adjacent organs). Thus, it is not surprising for a seemingly healthy individual to suddenly become diagnosed with MS during pregnancy. Pregnant patients with MS are not treated unless there are active/ongoing symptoms. The best approach to managing pregnant patients with MS is to medically treat with Diuretics and defer surgery until week 28 of pregnancy.

In general, there will be shortness of breath, as is the case for most symptomatic valvular disorders. Alternatively, the SOB can be present within the context of pulmonary edema. MS patients may develop a compensatory left atrial enlargement (in response to an underlying "stenosis"). An enlarged left atrium (visible as "notching" on EKG + "elevated left main bronchus" on CXR) places unnecessary pressure on the surrounding pulmonary vessels. The build up of pressure from within the pulmonary vessels (exacerbated via coughing) can lead to an increase in shearing forces, and therefore, hemoptysis (the act of coughing up blood). As the left atrium continues to enlarge in size (and the valve continues to constrict, respectively), the patient becomes susceptible to thromboembolism. Now, in the later stages of mitral stenosis, the patient is at elevated risk for atrial fibrillation (an indication for surgical repair). The weight of the atrium lifts the left main bronchus. In unusual cases, there can be concomitant paralysis of the recurrent laryngeal nerve (from an enlarging left atrium that exerts pressure on adjacent structures). This, in turn, leads to hoarseness.

As you can see, there is an elegant overlap between form and function. We've mentioned how there is elevated pressure within pulmonary vessels (in response to left atrium enlargement). The situation is particularly problematic if the patient ends up with Pulmonary HTN (an indication for surgical repair)

Treatment (definitive): **Mitral Valve Repair or Mitral Valve Replacement**

Aortic Regurgitation (AR)

Any condition that effectively compromises the structural integrity of the aortic valve may lead to AR. We have mentioned earlier that endocarditis has a role in the development of MR; the same can be said for endocarditis and AR. HTN is an independent risk factor for AR; patients with aortic dissection also have a history of HTN. Aortic dissection is a process that greatly dilates the annulus of the aortic valve. In other words, it makes the valve "floppier" or more "insufficient". Ehler's Danlos syndrome patients are at increased risk for dilatation of the ascending aorta. Likewise, other disorders with innate structural (e.g. connective tissue) deficiencies such as Marfan's syndrome may develop AR. Moreover, AR is associated with congenital bicuspid valve, SLE and ankylosing spondylitis.

Treatment (definitive): **Aortic Valve Repair or Aortic Valve Replacement**

Aortic Stenosis (AS)

When we discussed MS, it was mentioned that there was left atrium enlargement (in response to the stenosis at the level of the mitral valve). Likewise, for patients with AS, there is a left ventricular enlargement (in response to the stenosis at the level of the aortic valve). An EKG will demonstrate the presence of left ventricular hypertrophy (LVH).

Treatment (definitive): **Aortic Valve Replacement (not repair)**

*Myxomatous degeneration is defined as a condition in which the valve's connective tissue constituents have been compromised. Myxomatous is derived from the root myxo or 'mucus' or 'slime' – a good visual depiction of a loss of structural integrity. The valve is floppy or wide, potentially paving the way for mitral insufficiency.

Congenital Heart Disease

A congenital cyanotic heart disease entails an overall DECREASE in blood flow. Deoxygenated blood makes its way into the systemic circulation (by means of bypassing the lungs - the lungs is where you pick up oxygen). Cyanotic conditions are associated with underlying anatomical deficits (e.g. right-to-left shunting, great arterial mishaps). There may even be bidirectional shunting, resulting in an admixture of blood flow. Furthermore, communication between the chambers of the heart (or, transposition of great arteries) will lead to an INCREASE in pulmonary (vascular) resistance (PVR). The patient may appear visibly blue.

In contrast, a congenital acyanotic (non-cyanotic) heart disease entails an INCREASE in pulmonary blood flow. There is some degree of shunting (left-to-right), which manifests as the signs and symptoms of respiratory or circulatory compromise (e.g. tachypnea, shortness of breath, fatigue, etc.). The patient will generally exhibit normal blood oxygen levels.

Congenital Heart Disease (Acyanotic/Non-Cyanotic)

I. Atrial Septal Defect (ASD)

The majority of ASD pose negligible issues for patients, as the congenital heart defect is minor. In unusually rare cases, a right-to-left shunt may be associated with an increasing number of complications. ASD is an acyanotic condition.

II. Ventricular Septal Defect (VSD)

VSD is another acyanotic condition; it is the most common congenital heart defect, comprising roughly a quarter of all such lesions. VSD are generally asymptomatic and self-limiting. However, if the lesion is of sufficient size and left untreated, the patient may risk developing heart failure and/or failure to thrive.

III. Patent Duct Arteriosus (PDA)

PDA is a USMLE favorite, appearing on Step I, II, and III
Familiarize yourself with the murmur. There's a YouTube clip by *Thinklabs* available online.

Okay, now that you've listened to a simulation of a continuous machine-like murmur, don't miss it on the exam!

To be fair, most vignettes that support headphones can be answered directly from the information presented in the question. If you can recognize PDA from the vignette itself, you can save time by ignoring the headphone aspect of it.

What are the risk factors for developing PDA?

- A preterm birth event; a preterm status is non-specific and is associated with a myriad of conditions
- Family history of cardiac defects (not just PDA) or genetic defects (not just cardiac)
- High-altitude birth event (low-yield as far as the exams are concerned)
- Maternal rubella infection (generally in 1rst trimester or between week 1-12) -> PDA of the infant (the pathophysiology involves placental spread of the virus into the infant's circulatory system; the heart along with associated vessels are compromised)

a. PDA (uncomplicated)

Prevention (before the fact):

Vaccinations in the mother can prevent the development of Congenital Rubella Syndrome and therefore, PDA in the newborn. PDA is found in half of all infants with Congenital Rubella Syndrome.

Treatment (after the fact):

Patients with uncorrected PDA are at increased risk of developing heart failure as an adult. Administer NSAIDs (e.g. Indomethacin or Ibuprofen) in order to close the patent (opening).

b. PDA + Transposition of Great Vessels

Administer a prostaglandin to keep the Ductus Arteriosus (DA) open long enough to undergo surgical correction.

Congenital Heart Disease (Cyanotic)

I. Transposition of Great Vessels

In normal hearts, the aorticopulmonary septum develops in a spiraling manner (as opposed to Transposition of Great Vessels where it assumes a linear course)

Treatment: Surgical correction at birth (compare with Tetralogy of Fallot where the patient can still survive onto early childhood without surgical repair)

II. Tetralogy of Fallot

As the name suggests, there are 4 anatomical deviations that produce this condition, namely:

1. Stenosis of the pulmonary infundibulum
2. Overriding aorta
3. VSD
4. RVH

There is an observable sequence of clinical events that can be summarized as such:

VSD -> RVH-> ["tet spells" or "colic"] -> cyanosis -> loss of consciousness

In order to alleviate this sequence of events, the child may attempt squatting. What is the purpose of the squatting? The squatting maneuvers temporarily reverse the Right-to-Left shunt that leads to the cyanotic condition. It decreases the overall magnitude of the shunt.

Treatment: Surgical correction during early childhood (generally)

Don't get these two cyanotic conditions mixed up. Classically, the Transposition of Great Vessels patient will be a neonate and the Tetralogy of Fallot patient will be young child (e.g. age 2 or 3). Of course, this condition is not exclusive to children and adults with Tetralogy of Fallot may present with clubbing of the extremities (of the digits), indicating systemic manifestations. Radiological assessment necessary for diagnosis includes an echocardiogram. A deviant *"coeur-en-sabot"* (like a boot) shaped heart is visible on a CXR.

III. Ebstein Anomaly

Not a high yield topic. You can skip this section if you are pressed for time. Ebstein anomaly is associated with tricuspid regurgitation (TR). TR questions are uncommon on the exam, unless presented within the context of an IVDA patient. In short, the Ebstein anomaly is presented as another cyanotic, congenital heart disease that may lead to right-sided heart failure (if uncorrected).

Anatomically,

The right atrium predominates (hypertrophies) -> right ventricle shrinks ("atrialization" or atrophy) -> right heart failure and associated conduction abnormalities (e.g. Wolff Parkinson White Syndrome, right bundle branch block etc.)

Chapter 4: Miscellaneous Heart Diseases

Coarctation of the Aorta

As far as the exam is concerned, this condition is primarily found in girls   with Turner's syndrome or 45 XO karyotype. The best way to visualize this condition (as it relates to a Turner's syndrome female patient) is to consider the top half of the body as hypertensive. In order to apply this heuristic, we have to picture the bottom half of the body as hypotensive.

a. Hypertensive Component

- Notched ribbing indicates an increase in collateral circulation. In other words the vasculature has been ramped up to such a degree that it is literally leaving behind a physical imprint (scalloping) on ribs as per CXR. Of course, increased vessels/"circuitry" can be interpreted as an increase in blood pressure. More vessels are being recruited to keep up with the demands of the upper half of the body. This is a compensatory reaction to the coarctation (essentially, a narrowing of the aorta).
- A systolic murmur emanates from the back region
- Arterial hypertension of the arms (HTN of the upper extremities)

b. Hypotensive Component

- Low femoral pulse is evident

- Radio-femoral delay; normally there should not be a gap in radial and femoral pulsations. As discussed earlier, an imbalance exists between the upper and bottom half of the body.
- Lower extremities are cold with concomitant claudication (e.g. patient may complain of leg cramps). Claudication is generally due to obstruction of arteries or coarctation in the Turner's syndrome patient

When you are preparing for the Step 3 CCS exam*, you may encounter a practice case on Turner's syndrome. It is a comprehensive case that encompasses a myriad of tests: CBC, BMP, ultrasound of the abdomen and kidneys, X-ray of left wrist (evaluate for growth and development) echocardiogram, audiometry, karyotype analysis (genetic consult), gyn consult (e.g. streak ovaries and infertility) bone/skeletal survey (evaluate for growth and development), thyroid function tests (e.g. TSH), hemoglobin A1c (or fasting glucose level), BUN, creatinine, LH, FSH, LFTs, and psychiatric consult (to rule out developmental delay).

*A Turner's syndrome case should be available in the UWorld CCS software program that includes both interactive and read-out cases. The program provides further details on how to navigate the case on the exam, including sequence of orders and follow-up therapeutic and monitoring protocols, patient support or education/reassurance, consults etc. If you are in need of additional CCS training materials (for other topics aside from Turner's syndrome), Archer's review offers CCS worships. You also have access to prerecorded workshops. It is best to purchase CCS workshop recordings from the last 1 or 2 years as the format of the exam is always changing (despite being standardized in nature). Lastly, don't forget to practice with NBME software cases for the CCS.

Turner's syndrome can also present with bicuspid aortic valves.

Chapter 5: Coronary Artery Disease

You should be very comfortable with this topic. CAD (Coronary Artery Disease) or Ischemic Heart Disease is extremely high-yield because of the disease prevalence in the general population. The name coronary artery disease reflects its pathophysiology—the culprit being atherosclerosis of the arteries (of the cardiovascular system) or deposition of fibro-fatty plaques within the arterial wall. A third heart sound (S3) auscultated on physical exam is suggestive of dilated left ventricle. Likewise, a fourth heart sound (S4) auscultated on physical exam is suggestive of LVH.

Clinically, patients tend to conflate symptoms of CAD with GERD as they have superficial similarities (and sometimes, overlapping symptoms, e.g. atypical MI). It is for this reason that undiagnosed GERD is treated with the same care and level of urgency as CAD. In the exam, you are expected to run the same gamut of tests until acid reflux has been effectively ruled out. If you suspect GERD in the CCS, do not order esophageal pH monitoring, as it is regarded as an unnecessary, possibly invasive, investigation for the initial encounter.

Angina (stable and unstable) and myocardial infarctions (STEMI, NSTEMI) revolve around the principle of atherosclerosis. However, Prinzmetal/variant/vasospasm angina exhibits a different mechanism of action than other CADs. Keep in mind that variant angina does not share the same set of risk factors as angina or MI. Patients tend to be younger. No one has pinpointed the reason for variant angina (there are some hypotheses in circulation) but "vasospastic" conditions (e.g cocaine-induced MI, esophageal vasospasm,

Raynaud's etc.) seem to exhibit some overlapping patterns and characteristics. The only risk factor in common with other CVD is smoking.

Let's review general risk factors for CAD:

- Smoking (the practice negatively impacts vessels of all types and has the potential to exacerbate vessel damage in diabetics)
- Pertinent family history
- HTN (uncontrolled HTN, in and of itself, compromises the structural integrity of vessels)
- Obesity (usually goes hand-in-hand with serum LDL concentrations or high blood triglycerides; HDL exerts a protective effect)
- Diabetes (vessel and nerve damage are common in DM patients); DM is the most deleterious (of all risk factors)
- Sedentary lifestyle

These risk factors are almost never found in isolation; there is an overwhelming tendency for co-occurrence (comorbidity), which further compounds the problem. In order to minimize negative disease sequelae, preventative measures are always ideal.

Describe the pain symptoms of CAD?

- Substernal, chest pain (or chest discomfort); if he/she can pinpoint the pain/discomfort, then it suggests a different etiology (e.g. costochondritis, musculoskeletal etc.) as the sensation (e.g. tightness/pressure) tends to be somewhat "diffuse" or indistinct by nature
- Pain is alleviated by rest (angina) or not at all (MI)

- Pain is exacerbated by physical activity and/or the presence of emotional stressors (angina); this is not necessarily the case with MI where the culprit is a blocked coronary artery
- Pain emanates to other regions beyond the chest, notably, the shoulder, arm, jaw or neck (angina or MI)
- Pain associated with stable angina typically resolves in only a manner of minutes. In contrast, unstable angina and MI pain is present in excess of a half hour. Anything beyond 24 hours suggests a different etiology [e.g. costochondritis (tenderness is elicited), GERD, musculoskeletal etc.]

Pain that varies according to respiration has a pulmonary origin (with the exception of Pericarditis –Pericarditis is also affected by body position)

Keep in mind that not all patients conform to the expected patterns of pain for CAD (e.g. women, elderly and diabetics). These patients may experience atypical symptoms (e.g. flushing, diaphoresis, dyspnea, fatigue, excessive sweating etc.) or "silent" MI. It is important for the clinician to review diagnostic and investigative procedures within the context of risk factors.

Generally, cases involving a cardiac origin entail testing with EKG + CXR (order together on CCS). Confirmatory testing includes an ultrasound of the heart (i.e. echocardiogram/echocardiography/echo). A particular type of echo (e.g. transthoracic echocardiogram or TTE) is the underlined initial procedure of choice for investigating valvular issues (e.g. MR, MS, AR and AS), but CAD patients usually undergo testing with generic echocardiogram.

If the patient is stable and not currently experiencing an acute crisis, schedule a stress test. Never conduct a stress test when the patient is experiencing angina or MI (e.g. increases risk of sudden death or negative sequelae). Stress test is available in two "flavors", exercise and pharmacological (medication). COPD/asthma patients may be poor candidates for exercise stress test (e.g. SOB). However, testing via dobutamine administration is permissible in these conditions. Patients that are poor candidates for exercise stress testing (e.g amputees, feet ulcers, COPD, metabolic syndrome etc.) can partake in adenosine thallium or sestamibi scintigram studies (i.e. metabolic syndrome).

Let's review the exercise stress test. The Bruce Protocol measures cardiac activity and function during a treadmill exercise test. The USMLE may gauge your understanding of exercise stress test factors that portend negative outcomes. The Bruce Protocol has determined that a > 2 mm ST depression that is maintained for ≤ 6 minutes is indicative of severe cardiac compromise. The exam is notorious for presenting answer choices that are very close to what you remember. The signs may be switched around (<2 mm ST depression instead of the appropriate metric, > 2mm ST depression). They may try to throw you off by changing some of the cutoffs or even substituting "ST depression" with "ST elevation". Be mindful of the metrics that constitute negative prognostic factors – actually, be mindful of any portion of the exam that deals with criteria (e.g. diagnostic procedures, Ranson's etc.). However, if you've memorized about 2/3rd of these lists, you should be fine – you could simply deduce the answer by eliminating obvious wrong answer choices and/or distractors).

What are the untoward prognostic factors found on a stress test? (Memorize)

- ST elevation (ST elevation of any kind suggests a positive stress test)
- Low Blood Pressure (with respect to baseline)
- Heart Rate that falls below 70% of age-predicted maximal HR

- ST depression > 2mm (In general, a 1+ ST depression is enough for a positive stress test, but a 2mm+ ST elevation is indicative of severe CAD and has prognostic ramifications)

Untoward prognostic factors -> angiography

If the patient is done with his/her exercise testing session:

And, he/she maintains ST depression > 5 minutes -> angiography

Ambiguous stress testing results -> nuclear testing (this study is great for identifying the locus of ischemia or differentiating ongoing ischemia from previous infarctions/lesions)

Angina (stable)

As a disease entity, angina pectoris is related to MI. The patient experiences chest pain or discomfort (e.g. crushing/squeezing/tightness/choking/pressure etc.) as a function of activity or exertion. Symptoms subside when the patient is at rest. A clue on the exam – upon administration of S/L Nitroglycerine, the symptoms (i.e. chest pain/discomfort) resolve. Clinically speaking, angina is analogous to intermittent claudication. In short, it is "intermittent claudication of the chest".

It is not unusual for an EKG to yield normal or baseline findings. If chest pain/discomfort is evident, EKG *may* yield ST depression (similar to NSTEMI). Further diagnostics (e.g. EKG, exercise stress test, cardiac markers) may be warranted if there is reason to suspect underlying MI (rule out NSTEMI).

Prevention:

Lifestyle changes (modulate HTN, HLD*, smoking etc.), S/L nitroglycerine (prophylaxis)

Treatment **(acute crisis or event):**

S/L nitroglycerine is regarded as the initial therapy and will resolve the "claudication" by expanding the blood vessels; nitroglycerine is a vasodilator. The intervention is diagnostic, as symptom resolution will confirm underlying angina.

Treatment/Maintenance **(chronic angina):**

Aspirin* (or Clopidogrel) + Long Acting Nitrate Preparations (e.g. Isosorbide preparations) + Beta Blockers (BB)

If the patient has HLD, treat the cholesterol and/or high triglycerides, as well.

If the patient also has comorbid COPD/asthma or persistent slow Heart Rate, substitute Beta Blockers with Calcium Channel Blockers (CCB); CCB is the mainstay of treatment for patients with Variant angina.

If the patient has untoward prognostic factors (e.g. ST depression > 2mm) -> heart cath (angiogram/angiography are all acceptable and equivalent answer choices)

Angina with comorbid AS -> heart cath (angiogram/angiography are all acceptable and equivalent answer choices)

*Aspirin has a mortality benefit. Any medication or procedure with associated mortality benefit is given precedence in the exam

*In order to prevent Hyperlipidemia (HLD) in patients, statin therapy is initiated in healthy patients with LDL levels of 130 or higher. The cutoff is different for patients with a relevant history of CAD (or claudication), namely, start therapy at LDL levels that exceed 100. Because of the potential for vessel damage, DM patients with comorbid CAD symptoms should continue statin treatment to maintain LDL levels below 70.

Peripheral Arterial Disease (PAD) or Peripheral Vascular Disease (PVD) is analogous to angina in that there is pain, albeit, in the limbs, upon exertion or activity. Aside from pain symptoms, there is pallor (as well as "shininess") and inhibited pulses in the lower extremities. Additionally, there is an emphasis on preventative lifestyle changes (e.g. lipid management, smoking cessation, diabetic control etc.). The initial investigative technique is Ankle Brachial Index (ABI>1 is baseline). ABI is a high-yield test answer choice. It is preferred over other modalities due to convenience (accessibility) and cost-effectiveness. Of course, the gold standard would be Angiography, but it is generally not used, unless there is some element of ambiguity (instead, we use ultrasound to confirm diagnosis). There is a hierarchy of medical management:

Aspirin (Clopidogrel) >Cilostazol > Pentoxifylline [it is a rheological (rhéō ="flow") modulator and supposedly influences blood viscosity—sounds fancy, but it really doesn't do all that much; not the best answer choice by any means]

When symptomatology is evident upon rest (analogous to unstable angina) or becomes progressive in nature, recommend a surgical consult.

Angina (unstable)

Exactly what the name suggests, unstable angina is an *evolving* angina. It can be completely new; new onset angina that has persisted for at least 2 months (of duration) – the angina is in a state of flux (and therefore, unstable) –it is extreme and there are at least 3 events per day.

Alternatively, the angina is present during rest (devoid of activity or exertion). Any angina (with the exception of variant) that is active during rest is by definition, unstable. Angina at rest is always unstable.

Thirdly, a patient may have a history of angina (stable) that has evolved/progressed into angina (unstable). If there is a change in frequency/intensity/duration of angina events, the patient's angina (stable) is now reclassified as angina (unstable).

It is not unusual for an EKG to yield normal or baseline findings. If chest pain/discomfort is evident, EKG *may* yield ST depression (similar to NSTEMI). Stable and Unstable angina may yield a normal EKG or ST depression. In contrast, variant angina may yield ST elevation during an acute episode in which chest pain/discomfort is present. It is best to visualize angina (unstable) as a precursor to NSTEMI (both CADs may have ST depression on EKG) even if it doesn't progress into NSTEMI.

The therapeutic measures for unstable angina and NSTEMI are identical, as far as the exam is concerned.

Treatment of Unstable Angina

Oxygen + S/L Nitroglycerine + Aspirin + Clopidogrel + Heparin +Glycoprotein Receptor Antagonist Antagonist [(+/- Percutaneous Coronary Intervention (PCI*)]

Treatment of NSTEMI

Oxygen + S/L Nitroglycerine + Aspirin + Clopidogrel +Heparin +Glycoprotein Receptor Antagonist [(+/- Percutaneous Coronary Intervention (PCI)]

PCI includes PTCA (percutaneous transluminal coronary **angioplasty)– understand the sequence –intervention is predicated upon severity of risk factors. Angioplasty has a mortality benefit. If there is persistent chest pain in MI patients (NSTEMI or STEMI), you first perform a cardiac cath (the equivalent of an angiogram/angiography). After a cath has been completed, there are other options, including PTCA (angioplasty) or CABG (Coronary Artery Bypass Graft). "Graphy" precedes "Plasty". PCI is performed within the first 90 minutes of arrival at the hospital. Clopidogrel accompanies stenting and PTCA (angioplasty). Clopidogrel has a mortality benefit. Moreover, glycoprotein receptor antagonists and heparin have a mortality benefit. If given a choice during the exam between heparin and I.V LMW heparin, go with I.V LMW heparin; it is the preferred agent because there is no need for monitoring of anticoagulant effects. The most common adverse effect is uncontrolled bleeding. LMW heparin is also associated with Heparin Induced Thrombocytopenia (i.e. a drastic drop in platelet count). How do you reverse the effects of LMWH? Administer Protomine.*

Oxygen and nitrates are comfort measures with no recognizable mortality benefit.

For the CCS, you can **add a Beta Blocker, ACEi (or ARB), and statin as discharge medications.** They are an important part of the therapeutic management of MI patients. It is not necessary to include them in the initial set of orders for suspected MI patients.

Furthermore, patients should continue to use aspirin as part of their daily medication intake. These drugs all confer a mortality benefit.

These meds have some untoward effects, but the benefit outweighs the risks. If adverse effects emerge (e.g. cough or angioedema), the clinician could substitute ACE inhibitors with ARB. On rare occasions, ACEi and ARBs may be associated with hyperkalemia; potassium derangements (hyper and hypo) correspond with muscle problems (e.g. cramps, weakness, twitching etc.)

The use of Beta Blockers is associated with diarrhea, nausea, hypotension and sexual dysfunction. It can cause bronchospasms but is generally tolerable for most patients (including asthmatics and COPD). If possible, order cardio-selective (beta-1 receptor affinity) Beta Blockers in asthmatics and COPD patients. Order routine LFTs for patients that have been initiated on statin therapy; statin use is associated with elevated transaminases.

CABG is generally reserved for special cases:

(a) Left main coronary artery stenosis (> 70% occlusion)
(b) Triple-vessel compromise in asymptomatic patients
(c) Triple-vessel compromise in patients with angina (stable)
(d) Triple-vessel compromise in patients with poor ejection fraction (EF)
(e) Triple-vessel compromise in patients with proximal Left Anterior Descending (LAD) artery stenosis
(f) Double (or triple)-vessel compromise in patients with DM; DM is often regarded as a CHD risk equivalent and therefore the rationale for beginning CABG at the level of a diseased double vessel is quite understandable

How do you differentiate Unstable Angina from NSTEMI?

Cardiac enzymes (e.g. CK-MB and Troponin T) and biomarkers are underlined elevated in NSTEMI. The clinician orders cardiac enzymes x3 around every 7 hours to observe a decline in serum levels (for patients with unstable angina, order enzymes to rule out NSTEMI). If you suspect another MI event during the course of hospitalization, order CK-MB as it only rises for 2 days.

If time permits, please review the factors that determine a TIMI risk score. It isn't particularly high yield but will give you a better understanding of negative prognostic indicators of unstable angina.

Angina (Prinzmetal/variant/vasospasm)

This angina is a separate entity and exhibits a different mechanism of action than other CADs. Comorbid associations include, Raynaud's phenomena, aspirin-induced asthma and migraines. There is a female preponderance (middle-aged).

A cardiac cath or equivalent is performed (e.g. coronary angiography is the investigative technique of choice for suspected variant angina patients). The angiogram can be followed up with angioplasty, if the clinician deems it necessary. The purpose of the angiogram is to assess for the presence of spasms. If the spasms are not observed, but you strongly suspect a diagnosis of variant angina, perform a provocation test (to elicit vasospasms) – apply, Ergonovine (or Methylergonovine) challenge, acetylcholine or hyperventilation-induced testing.

Treatment **(acute crisis):**

S/L nitroglycerine

Treatment/Maintenance **(chronic variant angina):**

Calcium Channel Blocker*

*There is no role of beta-blockers in the treatment of variant angina. CCBs are effective in treating some forms of vasospasms (e.g. esophageal spasms, cocaine induced chest pain and Raynaud's phenomena)

Lastly, do not confuse diagnostic medications with treatment medications. The exam writers often scramble medications (diagnostic vs. treatment) for a number of disease entities – it is not unusual to see wrong answer choices that attempt to confuse prophylaxis with treatment, as per Migraine therapy, for example. Take home lessen: know the difference between diagnostic meds and treatment meds, prophylaxis and treatment, acute vs. chronic disease states (and the corresponding therapies).

Non–ST-segment elevation myocardial infarction (MI)

Let's review the basic description of MI. We have already touched upon some aspects of NSTEMI during our discussion about unstable angina. The bullet points are applicable to NSTEMI and STEMI.

- Chest pain (or chest discomfort); chest discomfort may be accompanied with SOB
- Pain is not alleviated by rest (as opposed to stable angina)
- Pain emanates to other regions beyond the chest, notably, the shoulder, arm, jaw or neck
- Pain is present in excess of a half hour
- +/- Flushing, diaphoresis, dyspnea, fatigue, excess sweating

Generally, cases involving a cardiac origin entail initial testing with EKG. Besides, an EKG will be necessary to differentiate NSTEMI from STEMI, as there is a difference in therapeutic management. Order cardiac enzymes. An X-ray can be ordered to rule out diseases with pulmonary manifestations. [In other cases with nebulous etiology, we order BNP to differentiate between diseases with pulmonary or cardiac origin (e.g. elevated BNP levels are found in CHF and/or ventricular dysfunction)].

Treatment of NSTEMI

Oxygen + S/L Nitroglycerine + Aspirin + Clopidogrel +Heparin +Glycoprotein Receptor Antagonist (+/- PCI)

For the CCS, memorize the trade name of at least one heparin medication and one glycoprotein receptor antagonist.

ST-segment elevation myocardial infarction (MI)

The basic description of MI still applies:

- Chest pain (or chest discomfort); chest discomfort may be accompanied with SOB
- Pain is not alleviated by rest (as opposed to stable angina)
- Pain emanates to other regions beyond the chest, notably, the shoulder, arm, jaw or neck
- Pain is present in excess of a half hour
- +/- Flushing, diaphoresis, dyspnea, fatigue, excess sweating

The main difference between STEMI and NSTEMI is the use of Thrombolytics. Thrombolytics is a mortality-lowering agent that is contraindicated in the treatment of NSTEMI

Treatment of STEMI

Thrombolytics (+/- PCI) +Oxygen + S/L Nitroglycerine + Aspirin + Clopidogrel +Heparin +Glycoprotein Receptor Antagonist

The exam gives you the choice of administering Thrombolytics or Angioplasty in patients with STEMI. If you've arrived in a large, nearby, urban facility (with "state-of-the-art" equipment), administer PCI/angioplasty, especially if you are within the **90-minute window**. If you've missed the window, go with Thrombolytics. The window for Thrombolytics is much longer (roughly **12-hour window**). Both forms of therapy confer a mortality benefit.

For the exam, know your contraindications. You don't have to memorize everything. For example, if you are confident in your understanding of the absolute contraindications for Thrombolytic therapy, you can skip memorizing the list of items that constitute the relative contraindications of Thrombolytic therapy. Why punish yourself? The exam tests your ability to efficiently navigate questions. You can often deduce the relative contraindications if you've already mastered understanding (or memory of) absolute contraindications, and vice versa. Also, know the cutoffs because they are also fair game for the test makers.

Absolute Contraindications for Thrombolytic Therapy:

- *Brain tumor*
- *Aortic dissection (latent)*
- *Ongoing (i.e. visible) bleeding/bleeding diathesis (and/or internal bleeding within past <u>6 weeks</u>)*
- *Head injury within past <u>3 weeks</u> (or brain surgery within past <u>6 months</u>)*
- *History of stroke within past <u>3 months</u>*

For the CCS, you can **add a Beta Blocker, ACEi (or ARB), and statin as discharge medications**. They are an important part of the therapeutic management of MI patients.

How do you differentiate NSTEMI from STEMI?

For all practical purposes, the symptoms are the same, but there will be ST elevation on EKG for STEMI, hence the name

How do you differentiate Angina (unstable) from MI?

Cardiac enzymes (e.g. CK-MB and Troponin) and biomarkers are <u>elevated</u> in a MI

Chapter 6: Heart Failure

An oversimplified schematic of heart failure posits that there are two types of heart failures. "Left"-sided heart failure and "Right"-sided heart failure –these models are based on the role of left and right ventricle with respect to heart supply. In actuality, there is a bit of a continuum that exists between both types of heart failures (in fact, a history of "L"-sided heart failure symptoms can precipitate "R"-sided heart failure). For the purpose of the exam, we should be able to differentiate "L"-sided heart failure from "R"-sided heart failure. S3 may be heard in patients with CHF or volume overload. S4 may be heard in CHF patients with diastolic component; patients with diastolic heart failure tend to have a long-standing HTN and/or diabetes.

"L"-sided heart failure

When you think of Left-sided heart failure, you should envision problems as systemic in nature, namely arising from the cardio-pulmonary circuit. In other words, the lungs and the heart are negatively affected by "L"-sided heart failure.

The symptoms of "L"-sided heart failure include:

- Edema of extremities (cardiovascular system; a CVS exam should yield pitting pedal edema)
- Dyspnea (cardiovascular system/pulmonary system)
- Orthopnea (pulmonary system; symptoms due to pulmonary congestion when the patient is lying down)

- Paroxysmal nocturnal dyspnea (PND) (pulmonary system; symptoms due to respiratory depression during sleep state; symptoms are pronounced in HF patients -> pulmonary congestion)
- Long-standing cough (primarily pulmonary system); night coughs can co-occur with PND

Physical Exam (Left-Heart Failure):

- Rales/crackles on auscultation
- S3 gallop
- Edema (pitting) on lower extremities

"R"-sided heart failure

When you think of Right-sided heart failure, you should envision problems that are somewhat less systemic in nature (unless, there is a pre-existing Left-sided heart failure). The liver is affected (e.g. hepatomegaly, positive hepatojugular reflux, congestive hepatopathy etc.). Yes, the pulmonary system is involved, albeit in a more decentralized manner than in "L"-sided heart failure. This is a probable sequence:

Pulmonary HTN -> *Cor Pulmonale* -> "R"-sided heart failure

Alternatively,

Pulmonary Stenosis -> *Cor Pulmonale* -> "R"-sided heart failure

When you think of "R"-sided heart failure, you think of... congestion, congestion and more congestion –this is due to backup of deoxygenated blood.

The symptoms of "R"-sided heart failure include:

- Edema of extremities, in particular, in the ankles (this is an example of "L"-sided heart failure -> "R"-sided heart failure); fluid build up or congestion in the ankles
- JVD (there is more congestion or fluid build up in "R"-sided heart failure); congestion in neck veins
- Fatigue (e.g. deoxygenated blood)

Physical Exam (Right-Heart Failure):

- Edema (pitting) on lower extremities with ankle edema
- JVD with hepatojugular reflux
- Hepatomegaly

Another distinguishing point – patients with "R"-sided heart failure may exhibit nocturia (usually within a context of PND) or an increase in urinary output (during the nighttime) in order to alleviate the congestion/build up of fluids. Patients with "L"-sided heart failure do not exhibit an increase in urinary output.

Prevention of Heart Failure: Lifestyle changes—address the comorbid conditions. If the patient has atrial fibrillation, administer rate control medications (patients with comorbid AF have increased mortality). Recommend substance abuse cessation if there is a pertinent history of alcohol, smoking and other substance use disorders (SUD). Address reversible causes of HF (e.g. thyrotoxicosis, HTN, anemia, etc.).

Also, regulate water and sodium intake. Encourage mild exercise routine. Avoid NSAIDs and Thiazolidinediones (e.g. Glitazones) as they exacerbate fluid retention in "high output" states.

Treatment of Heart Failure:

ACEi (or ARB) + Beta Blockers + Diuretic (e.g. Furosemide) + Spironolactone

Treatment of Heart Failure with Atrial Fibrillation:

ACEi (or ARB) + Beta Blockers + Diuretic (e.g. Furosemide) + Spironolactone + Digoxin

Treatment of Heart Failure with Anemia:

ACEi (or ARB) + Beta Blockers + Diuretic (e.g. Furosemide) + Spironolactone + parenteral iron

Treatment of Heart Failure with Pulmonary Edema:

Oxygen + Morphine + Nitrates + Diuretic (e.g. Furosemide)

Of the drug regimen for CHF, ACEi/ARB, Beta Blockers and Spironolactone (e.g. New York Heart Association class IV) confer a mortality benefit for the patient. Digoxin and Diuretics are NOT mortality-enhancing drugs, but are important for improving patient well-being by decreasing hospitalizations and the presence of comorbid symptoms.

Perhaps, you are wondering about the rationale for administering Beta Blockers in individuals with Heart Failure? It almost seems counterintuitive? Why would you want to slow down the heart in a patient suffering from Heart Failure? Evidence-Based Medicine from the past 40 years of clinical research strongly indicates the use of Beta Blockers in the treatment of Heart Failure. However, it has to be initiated at low doses and adequately titrated as such. Never initiate Beta Blocker therapy in acutely decompensated patients. If the heart needs an extra push (and there is issues concerning contractility or ejection fraction), consider augmenting the drug regimen with a positive inotropic agent (e.g. Dobutamine); Digoxin also exerts a positive inotropic effect on the heart.

Hypertropic Obstructive Cardiomyopathy (HOCM)

Another condition where it would seem counterintuitive to administer Beta Blockers is HOCM. Along with Diuretics, Beta Blockers are the drug of choice for the treatment of HOCM. HOCM is a USMLE favorite.

If you want to diminish the presence of murmurs upon auscultation (HOCM, MVP), implement the handgrip maneuver. In general, techniques that alleviate murmurs (upon auscultation) for HOCM and MVP have the exact opposite effect on other murmurs (e.g. MR, MS, AR and AS). And, amyl nitrate opposes that (e.g. exacerbates murmurs for HOCM and MVP). You're dealing with a whole lot of double negatives! Fortunately, the exam isn't too big on amyl nitrate. Squatting has the same effect as handgrip. Valsalva maneuver has the same effect as amyl nitrate.

Shortcut key:

Squatting=leg raise=handgrip -> treats (temporarily) murmurs for HOCM + MVP

Valsalva=standing=amyl nitrate=ACEi/ARB -> exacerbates (temporarily) murmurs for HOCM + MVP

The items in the above shortcut key have the opposite effect (with minor exceptions) on the other murmurs (e.g. MR, MS, AR and AS).

Why would you want to exacerbate a murmur?

It is a useful, diagnostic tool that helps the clinician confirm the suspicion of a murmur in the patient.

Treatment of HOCM:

Beta Blockers + Diuretics

What is a cause of sudden death in adolescents and young adults?

HOCM is often described in USMLE clinical vignettes of young, otherwise healthy individuals (often athletes)

What is a cause of sudden death in the elderly?

Aortic stenosis. AS is more commonly associated with angina, SOB and syncope. Valve replacement is the definitive treatment for patients with aortic stenosis.

Chapter 7: Rhythm Dysfunction

In general, for the purpose of the exam, patients that present with any form of heart block (e.g. 2ⁿᵈ and 3ʳᵈ degree heart block, left bundle branch block, bifascicular etc.), especially, within the context of an MI, are good candidates for pacemaker. Bradycardia is defined as adult heart rate that falls below 60 beats per minute; it is not treated unless the patient exhibits symptoms that are distressing. IV atropine is administered for patients with unstable bradycardia. As an anticholinergic/antimuscarinic, Atropine is used to treat slow HR. Naturally; we would expect fast HR to be one of the common side effects of Atropine use. In addition, Atropine shares the same side effects with other anticholinergics (e.g. urinary retention, dry mouth and pupillary dilation). However, if the patient presents with new onset MI and bradycardia, it is best to treat with a pacemaker. The definitive treatment for Tachy-Brady syndrome is installing a dual chamber pacemaker.

Tachycardia—

In this section, we are dealing with rhythms in the adult population. The cutoffs are completely different when applied to a newborn. The most common reason for tachycardia (HR> 100) is fever. This is a benign reflexive attribute and a physiological coping mechanism of the body. Aside from infections, there may be tachycardia in patients with vasculitis (i.e. inflammatory conditions), especially if the symptoms are new onset or acute in nature. Sinus tachycardia may be manifested in persons post-exercise or in response to a stressor (e.g. anxiety, potentially panic attacks). Pain symptoms are also associated with tachycardia. Reversible causes of tachycardia include hyperthyroidism, high-output HF, anemia and substance withdrawal.

Atrial Fibrillation (A-fib) —

Irregularly, irregular heart beats that progressively persists over time. Risk factors overlap with that of CAD. In many cases, the patient remains asymptomatic for quite some time. Patients with atrial fibrillation may exhibit the following symptoms:

- Palpitations (irregular beats/pulse may cause the patient to be subjectively aware of the muscle contractions from within the chest)
- Syncope (syncope can have a cardiac or neurological origin; cardiac arrhythmias may occur when the heart beats too rapidly or slowly
- SOB (dyspnea can either be of cardiac or pulmonary origin)
- Chest pain (there may be a sensation of pain that emanates from within the chest); patients with comorbid angina are more likely to experience chest pain

EKGs are the most important diagnostic modality for revealing information regarding arrhythmias. An EKG reading of a patient with atrial fibrillation will yield SVT (Supraventricular Tachycardia). In fact, atrial fibrillation is regarded as a subset of SVT. If you are unable to diagnose the patient via EKG (if patient is not symptomatic during the office visit or ER), assign the patient a Holter monitor. In addition, you will order TFT (to rule out reversible causes of atrial fibrillation) and echocardiogram to evaluate for the presence of clots.

Treatment of atrial fibrillation:

Beta Blockers (or Calcium Channel Blockers or Digoxin)

Treatment of atrial fibrillation + loss of consciousness:

Synchronized cardioversion

Treatment of atrial fibrillation + angina:

Synchronized cardioversion

Treatment of atrial fibrillation + BP <90:

Synchronized cardioversion

If time permits, please review the factors that determine a CHADS score. It isn't particularly high yield but will give you a better understanding of factors that dictate the appropriateness of anticoagulation therapy. For patients that are stable, cardioversion (electrical or medical) may be initiated before or after rate control; if acute crisis presents within two days of symptomatology, you may begin with cardioversion.

An acute crisis of atrial fibrillation necessitates I.V administration of therapeutics (e.g. I.V Diltiazem, I.V Heparin etc.) in order to ensure rapid delivery. Anticoagulation therapy can be initiated following a baseline echocardiogram.

Supraventricular Tachycardia (SVT)—

The symptoms are identical to that of atrial fibrillation, primarily because atrial fibrillation is a type of SVT.

Prevention (of SVT):

Digoxin; definitive (**ablation therapy**)

Treatment of SVT:

In many cases, conservative measures are enough to convert SVT to sinus rhythm. The **vagal maneuver techniques** include, unilateral carotid massage and valsalva. If these techniques fail, the clinician can implement medical management [e.g. **Adenosine (I.V), Beta Blockers, Calcium Channel Blockers or Digoxin**].

If a patient has been placed on Digoxin therapy as a preventative measure for SVT, there is a possibility for Digoxin intoxication. The vignette will describe the symptoms of excess Digoxin levels (e.g. <u>disturbances of color vision</u>). Digibind is the antidote for Digoxin intoxication. However, synchronized cardioversion is a contraindication in this particular situation (even if the patient demonstrates cardinal symptoms of hemodynamic instability – a loss of consciousness, systolic blood pressure < 90, heart failure and/or angina symptoms).

Cardioversion is safe during pregnancy (in general, electrical procedures, whether it be electrical cardioversion or ECT pose no problems during the course of pregnancy). However, Warfarin-based anticoagulation therapy is contraindicated during pregnancy; Warfarin is associated with fetal warfarin syndrome, skeletal deformities (e.g. nasal hypoplasia), limb defects, low birth weight and psychosocial effects.

The EKG of SVT is high-yield:

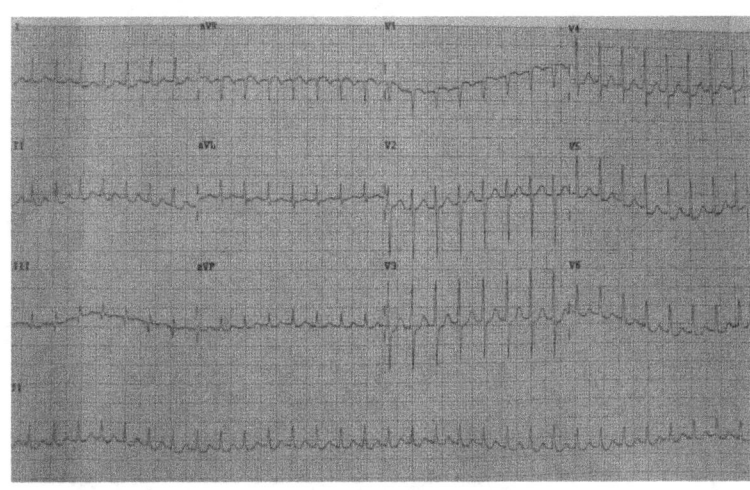

Atrial Flutter —

Atrial flutter (along with atrial fibrillation) is another type of SVT. The general guidelines for the medical management of atrial fibrillation and SVT also apply in patients with atrial flutter. Evaluate with echocardiogram to identify clot formation.

Treatment of atrial flutter:

Beta Blockers (or Calcium Channel Blockers or Digoxin)

The EKG of atrial flutter is high-yield and classic ("saw-tooth" pattern):

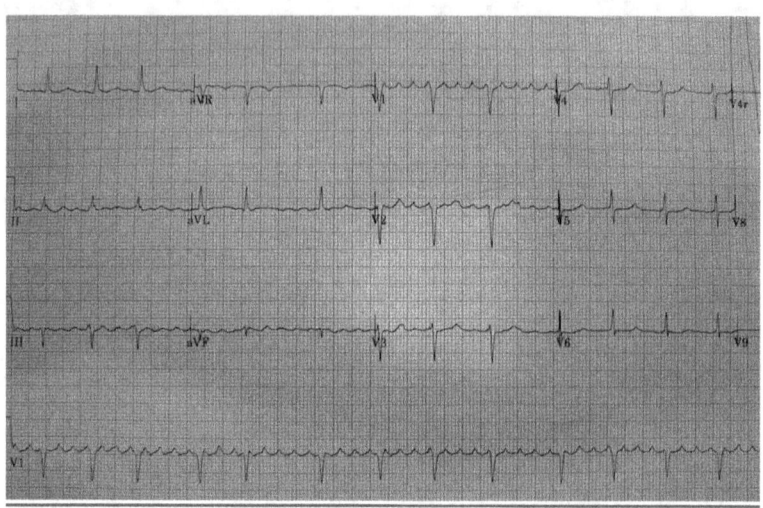

Multiform Atrial Tachycardia (MAT)—

We don't have to make this complicated. MAT= SVT + COPD (or asthma). Beta Blockers are contraindicated, probably because it exacerbates the underlying COPD symptoms. Oxygen is beneficial as it would be in patients with isolated COPD.

Wolff-Parkinson-White Syndrome (WPW)—

This is basically a variation of SVT that alternates with Ventricular Tachycardia (VT). If the patient has symptoms (e.g. dizziness and/or symptoms associated with SVT), the clinician may treat medically with <u>Procainamide.</u> However, it makes sense to sever the accessory pathway that creates a communication bridge between the atria and ventricles via <u>radiofrequency ablation</u>. The patient should stay away from any medication that slows down the heart's conduction system.

The EKG of WPW is high-yield (look for the characteristic <u>delta</u> <u>wave</u>):

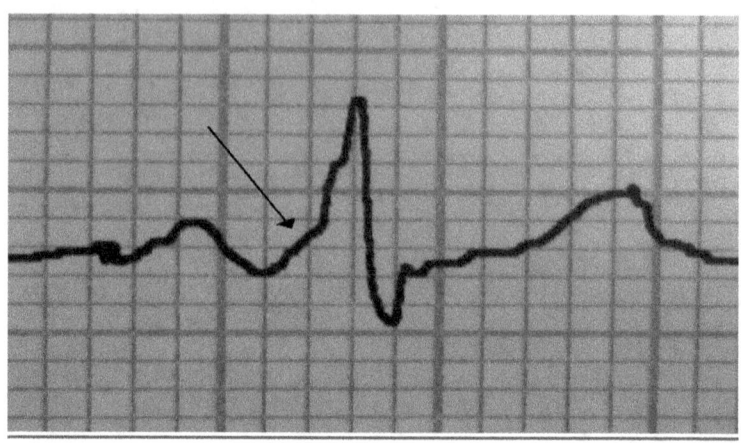

Ventricular Fibrillation (V-fib) —

CC: sudden death (note that Ventricular Tachycardia can also present with sudden death)

Treatment of V-fib: **UN**synchronized cardioversion. Don't bother doing anything else first, as it would be regarded as futility of treatment. However, there is a protocol:

(As per American Heart Association) Begin with CAB (e.g. CPR)

-> Unsynchronized cardioversion -> I.V Epinephrine -> Unsynchronized cardioversion -> I.V Amiodarone (alternatively, Lidocaine) -> Unsynchronized cardioversion

Cardioversion=Defibrillation

Don't just memorize, try to understand what is going on here. A debrillation device is used to DE-fibrillate (or, UN-fibrillate) a "fibrillating" condition. In other words, the clinician (or emergency personnel) will attempt cardioversion (defibrillation) procedures on conditions that require de-fibrillating, namely, A-fib and V-fib. However, there is an important difference. Synchronized cardioversion is used in patients with A-fib, while those with V-fib are treated with unsynchronized cardioversion.

Ventricular Tachycardia —

Patients that present with V-tach can be treated medically or electrically (e.g. hemodynamic instability)

Treatment of V-tach:

Amiodarone (or Procainamide)*

*If these answer choices are not available, try Lidocaine (not 1rst line). Furthermore, Magnesium can also be used to treat V-tach. However, the exam is more likely to associate Magnesium therapy with *Torsades de Pointes* (a variation of V-tach).

If the patient with V-tach is not particularly stable, cardioversion technique can be attempted (synchronized cardioversion). Do not use unsynchronized cardioversion –it is only indicated for treatment of V-fib.

The EKG of *Torsades de Pointes* is high-yield:

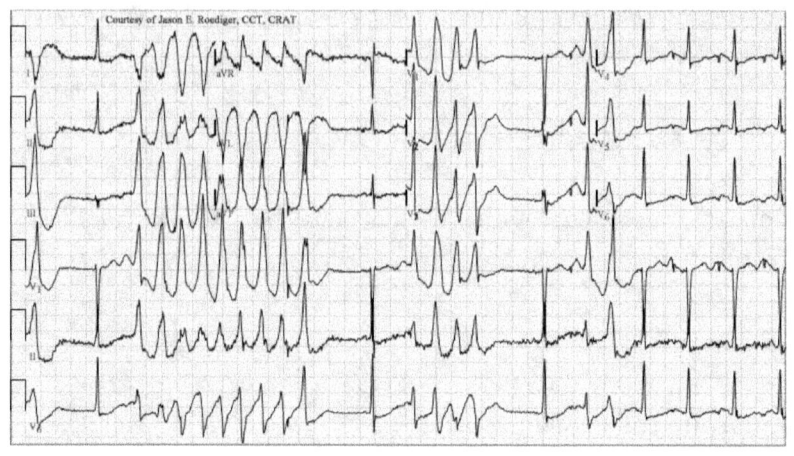

Chapter 8: Hypertension

As a rule, exam questions are prioritized in a manner that appropriately represents diagnosis found in the real world. HTN or essential HTN happens to be one of those topics that should be on the very top of every student's study list (along with MI and DM). Know your antihypertensive medications and respective side effects. Also, know about the preferred medications for a particular demographic (e.g. ACEi/ARBs) as well as the drugs that are given during the course of pregnancy (e.g. Labetalol, Methylprednisolone).

The exam covers mostly Primary HTN ("idiopathic" or "essential") but expects you to know about the less common 2ndary HTN. We've covered Coarctation of Aorta earlier in the notes. There is also Primary Hyperaldosteronism (there will be low renin levels), Pheochromocytoma (measure serum catecholamine and metanephrine or urine metanephrine), and Renal Artery Stenosis. HTN due to Renal Artery Stenosis has two variants, namely, Fibromuscular Dysplasia in children and middle-aged women, and Atherosclerosis (of renal arteries) in the elderly.

There is a classic presentation of HTN found in the CCS. Patient will come in for "wellness exam" or needs to undergo a physical evaluation in order to begin work or school. There may be a pertinent history of HTN in the family. Patient may have other risk factors for new onset HTN (e.g. sedentary lifestyle, lipid markers or sedentary lifestyle). Here is a probable sequence:

[Office visit] Patient has BP of 158/95 +/- slight obesity -> instruct lifestyle modification; high fiber, low salt diet, exercise program, +/- smoking cessation. Forward the clock by 6-8 weeks.

[Office visit 2] no significant changes. Forward the clock by 6-8 weeks.

[Office visit 3] no significant changes. Discharge patient with Hydrochlorothiazide P.O. Forward the clock by 6-8 weeks.

The patient begins Monotherapy with antihypertensive medication for his Stage I HTN (always, start with Hydrochlorothiazide unless it is contraindicated). Stage I HTN [140 to 159 mm Hg for systolic component and 90 to 99 for diastolic component]. A second drug can be added to the regimen if the patient progresses to Stage II HTN [160+ mm Hg for systolic component and 100+ mm Hg for diastolic component].

Know the difference between Hypertensive Urgency (180/110 + mm Hg with no prevailing symptomatology), Hypertensive Emergency (180/110 + mm Hg with systemic compromise; admit to ICU and initiate I.V therapeutic intervention), and Malignant HTN (Hypertensive Emergency +Papilledema); in order to prevent further end-organ damage, treatment should be titrated, accordingly.

Chapter 9: Abdominal Aortic Aneurysm & Aortic Dissection

Abdominal Aortic Aneurysm (AAA)–

Screening is performed for individuals with the following attributes:

65+ year old, male smoker

A pulsatile, abdominal mass is detected by ultrasound. Most commonly, the patient is asymptomatic. However, the patient may present with abdominal (pressure symptoms) or back pain (radiation); severe back pain represents rupture of AAA.

If the aortic arch is affected, there may be hoarseness from paralysis of recurrent laryngeal nerve.

An intact AAA patient may have a history of HTN. A **ruptured AAA** patient will present with **hypotension** (compare with aortic dissection patients that present with hypertension).

Treatment of Abdominal Aortic Aneurysm (AAA):

Beta Blockers

Treatment of Abdominal Aortic Aneurysm (AAA) of size 5cm +:

Surgical repair

Treatment of Abdominal Aortic Aneurysm (AAA) + Marfan's Syndrome (or Ehlers Danlos Syndrome):

Surgical repair

Therapy with Beta Blockers serves a dual purpose – it alleviates HTN symptoms in patients with intact AAA and prevents further growth of aneurysm.

Aortic Dissection—

Do not confuse with AAA. A ruptured AAA presents with Hypotension. Intact AAA patients are generally male, elderly smokers +/- HTN.

Aortic Dissection *always* presents with HTN, and in some cases Malignant HTN (treat with I.V antihypertensives). While patients with AAA may have risk factors such as Marfan's Syndrome (or Ehlers Danlos Syndrome), these attributes are far more common in patients with Aortic Dissections (as they contribute to the propagation of intimal tear).

A physical examination will yield asymmetric distribution of blood pressures. Remember, in the Turner's syndrome patient there were hypertensive (top) and hypotensive (bottom) components of the body. Except, in patients with Aortic Dissection, the right side of the body will be hypertensive and the left side of the body will be normotensive (or hypotensive). CXR of the body will reveal a "widening of the mediastinum" –this is a buzzword and diagnostic clue. There will also be an AR, which contributes towards maintaining an asymmetrical pulse.

Lastly, there are two types of Aortic Dissections. Type A is more serious and warrants surgical intervention as the site of the intimal tear is directly at the aortic arch. Type B Aortic dissection does not affect the arch and is generally managed by medications.

Treatment of Aortic Dissection, Type A:

Surgical Repair

Treatment of Aortic Dissection, Type B:

I.V Beta Blockers (to avoid recoil) + I.V antihypertensives (e.g. I.V Nitroprusside)

Conclusion

Thank you again for purchasing this book!

Remember, the exam is very doable! If you can handle medical school, you can certainly handle this exam. Stay away from negative people. If you exercise, continue exercising. Do not disrupt your daily routine. It isn't about how many hours you study in a given day, but how efficiently you study. Try to get in the mind of the test maker (whenever possible)! Take practice exams. Get plenty of sleep and do not stress! What's the point of unnecessary stress anyway? Do not think about vacations or imagine rewarding yourself...not until the exam is DONE! If you found this book helpful, please leave a positive review and/or comment. I am wishing you the very best! You can do it!

References

1. Harrison's Principles of Internal Medicine, 17th Edition

Appendix

<u>Efficient Test Taking Strategies</u>

1   Limit the number of sources for studying. A set of notes combined with one or two test banks is sufficient to master the exam. If you use multiple sources (e.g. 4 or more), you are more likely to run into contradictions. Not all exam preparation tools are updated at the same rate. There is also the very real possibility of running into a difference in opinion or judgment with respect to criteria (e.g. risk factors for ob-gyn cancers).

2   Master your notes. Personalize/customize your notes. Make your notes REAL and meaningful to you. The more intimate you get with the notes, the greater the chances of you internalizing the key concepts. Most test prep companies advise reading their notes a total of 3-5 times. Successive readings should be significantly faster than the previous. At least 1 or 2 readings should be exhaustive and detail oriented. Do a comprehensive wrap-up of all your core topics once every 2 weeks or so. The purpose of each reading is for retention. You might notice a few more details with your next read. Say, a certain protocol has a set of 10 criteria. Perhaps, you only got around to picking up 5 or 6 out of the 10 items during your 2nd or 3rd read. By the time you have finished your preparation, you will be even more comfortable with the material. The more factoids you pick up, the more likely you are to improve your ability to precisely select the correct answer choice (or rule out the less obvious distractor choice).

3   When in doubt, simplify your train of thoughts. Complex concepts can be broken down to easy, bite-size morsels of information.

4   Complete the test bank at least TWICE. Read and understand the commentary. Pay attention to any factoids presented in the question stem. Why did the test writer include a particular laboratory value? What information was purposely withheld (if any)?

5   Do not waste time on insets, graphs or tables. A lot of information might be presented to you at once in the vignette. Most of the time, you can skim graph or table-based vignettes by focusing on key concepts. Look at the last line of the vignette. What is the chief issue? What is the general trend in variables? Is X directly or inversely proportional to Y? Does the answer choice even make sense if you were not provided the vignette and accompanying tables, graphs or charts? If you are presented with a massive newspaper reprint in your question stem, do not read the whole thing. If you can identify a murmur simply by reading the vignette, then there is no point in equipping your headphones.

6   There are two ways of learning — visually, and by memorization. If you tend to learn exclusively by memory, try incorporating some visual techniques or thinking about things conceptually. If you have a habit of working out concepts, try to implement memorization techniques as well. This strategy will allow you to build up two separate memory systems, doubly reinforcing the overall learning process. If you happen to blank out on the day of the exam (or during practice exams or quizzes), you will have another method available at your disposal to work out the solution to the problem.

7   You have the option to memorize common laboratory values —I generally don't. It can, however, save you a few seconds

on the exam, especially if you have issues with finishing standardized exams on time.

8   Do not wrestle with questions. It's not personal. The test writers don't care if someone passes or fails. Never assume that they are intentionally trying to hold you back. Sometimes the very first question in a test section might be intimidating. We've all experienced that dreadful situation! Forget about it. Return to the question at a later point, if time permits. It's not worth jeopardizing the next three questions simply because you absolutely had to solve a particular question. Just don't. People have failed exams because they were stubborn about it.

9   Have sufficient sleep, whether it is 6 hours or 9 hours a day. Whatever works for you. Sleep allows you to perform your very best. Sleep is necessary for consolidating information and facilitates synaptic plasticity. Also maintain good sleep hygiene and a somewhat regular schedule.

10 Exercise about 3 times a week minimum. Exercise improves circulation to the brain and keeps you from zoning out during your study routine. If you aren't particularly active, walk outside for 20 minutes or so.

11 Do not think about vacations, video games and treating yourself until the exam is out of the way. Engaging in these indulgent thoughts will only serve to distract you. These ideations encourage you to lose your guard and become less disciplined during your preparation routine. Whenever these thoughts come to your head, block them out. Having said this, once you pass the exam, reward yourself BIG. You earned it!

12 Do not compare yourself to others, except in a positive light. Some folks have been studying all through medical school, perhaps, even secretly. Therefore, they might say, "I've only studied for 3 weeks using only question banks…and I've

scored 99%". People will say ridiculous things on the forums to throw others off. Do not take risks; be reasonable in your study preparation plan. Also, excellent question bank scores do not translate into excellent exam scores. NBME scores are a more reliable indicator for actual test performance, especially for Step 1 and 2 licensing exams.

13 Do not drag out your test preparation schedule. Taking 6 or 7 months to study for the exam will not yield superior scores. Step 1 or 2 should not take longer than 1.5 to 3 months. Step 3 preparation should be completed in less than 4 months max (Don't forget to factor in the CCS section of the exam! — it's not crammable)

14 Empty your mind. Avoid stressors. People tend to do well when there aren't life-changing issues in the background (e.g. divorces, custody battles, illnesses, deaths in the family etc.). Do not take the exam if you are dealing with a crisis…or, at the very least rent a motel or find an appropriate, distraction-free place to retreat to.

Images are licensed under Creative Commons, as per Wikipedia.

www.ingramcontent.com/pod-product-compliance
Lightning Source LLC
Chambersburg PA
CBHW051330220526
45468CB00004B/1578